WHEATGRASS DIET

Wheatgrass Diet: A Comprehensive Guide on Health Benefits, Nutrition, and Maintaining a Healthy Weight for Life

CHAD BRUNO

Table of Contents

Introductory

The term "wheatgrass diet" often refers to a dietary program that incorporates wheatgrass as a prominent component. Wheatgrass, or the tender, newly grown grass of the wheat plant Triticum aestivum, is a popular food and nutritional supplement.

Many people believe wheatgrass to be a superfood due to the high concentration of vitamins, minerals, antioxidants, and chlorophyll it contains. Proponents of the wheatgrass diet claim it can help with a variety of health issues, including detoxification, digestion, energy, and immunity.

Included in a wheatgrass diet plan could be:

• **Wheatgrass Juice:** its standard practice to drink freshly squeezed wheatgrass juice. This drink is commonly drunk on an empty stomach for its potential health advantages.

• Some choose to augment their diet with wheatgrass by taking wheatgrass pills or wheatgrass powder.

- Some people even put raw wheatgrass in their smoothies and salads.

It's worth noting that research backing up many of the purported benefits of the wheatgrass diet is scant and conflicting. Wheatgrass is healthy, but it's not meant to take the place of a varied and balanced diet, so it's best to drink it in moderation. If you have a history of medical issues or allergies, talk to your doctor before adding wheatgrass to your diet.

It's best to check with a doctor to be sure adding wheatgrass to your diet is safe and acceptable for your unique health and nutritional needs before making any major changes.

CHAPTER ONE
Benefits of Using Wheatgrass

Young Triticum aestivum shoots are sometimes referred to as "wheatgrass" since they are harvested at such a tender age. These tender new shoots have been called "superfoods" for their high nutrient content and potential health benefits. Some of the "power" and potential health advantages of wheatgrass are as follows:

• Wheatgrass has a high nutrient density, with vitamins A, C, and E, minerals iron, magnesium, calcium, amino acids, and enzymes all present in high concentrations. These nutrients play an important role in maintaining health and providing the body with the fuel it needs to thrive.

- Wheatgrass is brimming with chlorophyll, the green ingredient that gives plants their distinctive hue. Chlorophyll is a powerful antioxidant that may facilitate detoxification and lessen the effects of oxidative stress on the body.

- **Digestive Health:** Some proponents suggest that wheatgrass can enhance digestive health by increasing the function of the digestive tract, reducing bloating, and treating difficulties like constipation.

• Wheatgrass's minerals and antioxidants are thought to boost the immune system, making it better able to ward off infections and illnesses.

• Wheatgrass is widely used for its purported ability to increase energy and decrease weariness, however the supporting scientific evidence is scant.

• Wheatgrass is commonly touted as a detoxification aid due to claims that it helps flush out harmful substances like chemicals and metals from the body. However, the supporting research for these assertions is scant.

• Some research has linked wheatgrass' antioxidant and anti-inflammatory characteristics to its potential ability to fight cancer. More study is required, nevertheless, to verify these results.

• Wheatgrass juice or lotions applied topically are thought to alleviate skin issues such acne, eczema, and psoriasis.

• Wheatgrass' low calorie content and presumed capacity to promote weight control attempts have led to its inclusion in various weights loss regimens.

Wheatgrass is a popular dietary supplement because of its high nutrient and antioxidant content; however, many of the purported health benefits of wheatgrass are supported only by anecdotal evidence, and the results of scientific studies are inconsistent. In addition, some people may be allergic or experience negative side effects when consuming wheatgrass.

To be sure wheatgrass is safe and appropriate for your health needs, it's best to talk to a doctor before include it in your diet or utilizing it in any other way.

Consuming Wheatgrass to Improve Health

There are numerous approaches to adding wheatgrass to your diet. Wheatgrass is typically ingested in the form of a fresh juice, powder, or capsules. Some suggestions for eating wheatgrass:

1. Juicing Wheat Grass:

• Wheatgrass juice made from freshly harvested wheatgrass is one of the most popular ways to take in this superfood. You can find wheatgrass shots in juice bars, or you can cultivate and juice it at home with a wheatgrass juicer.

• To increase the health benefits of your smoothie, try adding some wheatgrass juice. Apples, oranges, and pineapples are some of the fruits that go well with it.

2. Wheat Grass Extract:

• Protein shakes and smoothies: add wheatgrass powder. Fruits, yogurt, and either dairy or soy milk can be added as well.

• Blend wheatgrass powder with water or your favorite fruit drink. Start with a little amount and gradually raise the dosage as your taste receptors adjust.

Wheatgrass powder can be used as a garnish or addition to salads.

3. Pills Made From Wheatgrass:

• Wheatgrass capsules and pills are available if the grass's flavor puts you off. The health benefits of wheatgrass are here, without the unpleasant aftertaste.

4. Wheatgrass Juice:

• Wheatgrass shots, which can be purchased in some health food stores and juice bars, are a convenient way to get a concentrated dose of the plant's nutrients all at once.

5. Recipes for Making Your Own Wheatgrass:

• You're free to use your imagination and try out new recipes. Popsicles, energy bars, and homemade salad dressings are just some of the creative ways that wheatgrass can be used.

6. Tasses de wheatgrass:

• Tea made from dried wheatgrass and heated water is called wheatgrass tea. This is a less usual way to eat it, but it can be a gentler experience.

You should know that the taste of wheatgrass can be rather strong and grassy, and it may take some time to get used to. If you've never tried wheatgrass before, ease into it by consuming only a small amount at first. Some people may feel stomach pain or other negative effects, so it's important to pay attention to your own body and make sure it's okay with what you're doing.

You should also consult a medical professional before making any significant dietary changes, including the addition of wheatgrass, especially if you have any preexisting health conditions or are taking any medications, as wheatgrass may interact with these substances or cause allergic reactions in some people.

CHAPTER TWO
Plan For A Wheatgrass-Based Diet

Unlike the ketogenic, Mediterranean, or vegetarian diets, the wheatgrass diet plan does not adhere to any strict dietary guidelines. Instead, you can try adding wheatgrass, which is the grass-like first growth of the wheat plant, to your regular diet. An example wheatgrass eating regimen is provided below.

• Eat a little wheatgrass every day. Wheatgrass is available in many different preparations, including juice, powder, and capsules. Your tastes and health objectives will determine the quantity and frequency.

• Wheatgrass juice for breakfast:

Wheatgrass shots, consisting of a tiny amount of freshly squeezed wheatgrass juice, are a popular way to kick off the day for many. This is commonly drunk first thing in the morning.

• Blended Wheatgrass Beverages:

Supplement your morning smoothie with a serving of wheatgrass juice or powder. To make a healthy and filling breakfast, add some fruit, vegetables, yogurt, or anything else you like.

• Munchable Wheatgrass:

Wheatgrass is a healthy addition to any snack. It's a great ingredient for homemade energy bars, yogurt, and salads.

• Dinner and Lunch:

Keep adding wheatgrass to your diet, either as a salad dressing or, if you find suitable recipes, as an ingredient in your main dishes.

• Wheatgrass for Hydration:

To stay hydrated and reap wheatgrass powder's nutritional

benefits, try mixing it with water or your preferred beverage.

• Dietitian or nutritionist consultation:

Consult a dietitian or nutritionist before beginning a wheatgrass diet if you are doing so for medical reasons. They can tailor a diet to your specific requirements and interests in order to help you achieve your health objectives.

• Keep an Eye on Your Health:

Maintain a record of your progress toward your health goals while on the wheatgrass diet. Keep track of any shifts in your vitality, digestion, and overall health.

• **Add to a Healthy Diet:**

Keep in mind that wheatgrass is meant to supplement a healthy diet, not to replace it. Continue eating a wide range of foods to ensure you're getting enough of everything your body needs.

• **Keep Allergies and Adverse Effects in Mind**

Wheatgrass may cause allergic reactions or side effects like nausea or gastrointestinal distress in some people. If you experience any negative side effects, you should stop using the product immediately.

• **Avoid Dehydration:**

Wheatgrass can have a mild diuretic effect; therefore, it is important to drink plenty of water when consuming it.

• **Preserve Contrast:**

Variety is key to a healthy diet. Wheatgrass is great, but it shouldn't be your only source of nutrition. Include a variety of fresh produce, whole grains, lean proteins, and heart-healthy fats in your diet.

The wheatgrass diet plan can be altered to suit the needs and goals of each individual. Wheatgrass is a nutrient-dense food, but the scientific evidence supporting many of its purported health benefits is scant. Consult with a healthcare professional or a registered dietitian before making significant dietary changes to ensure that the wheatgrass diet is suitable for your specific health needs.

Slimming Down With Wheatgrass

Wheatgrass's low calorie count and potential nutritional benefits have made it a popular weight loss supplement. Wheatgrass can be useful as part of a weight loss strategy, but it shouldn't be seen as a panacea on its own. Diet, exercise, lifestyle choices, and genetics all play a role in weight loss success.

Possible links between wheatgrass and slimming down are as follows:

• **Low in Calories:** Wheatgrass is low in calories but high in nutrients. Including it in your diet can help you cut back on calories, making it simpler to keep up with the calorie deficit that you need to lose weight.

• Wheatgrass is nutrient-dense, meaning it provides vitamins, minerals, and antioxidants despite having a low calorie content. It's a great way to get the nutrients you need without overdoing it on calories.

• **Detoxification:** Some proponents claim that wheatgrass can help with detoxification by promoting the removal of toxins and waste from the body. Even though there isn't a ton of proof that detox diets work, a properly functioning detoxification system can help you lose weight by enhancing your metabolism and digestion.

• Some people have found that ingesting wheatgrass helps them keep their hunger at bay and decreases their desire for unhealthy snacks. Weight loss and reduced caloric intake may result from this.

• Wheatgrass is rumored to give you more pep in your step, which means you can get more exercise in and thus burn more calories.

• There Is No Miracle Cure: Consuming only wheatgrass will not result in noticeable weight loss. It's important to incorporate it into a well-rounded diet and way of life.

• When trying to lose weight, it's important to eat a diet that's both varied and moderate in calories and other nutrients. The basic tenets of weight loss are a decrease in calorie intake and an increase in physical activity.

• **Exercising:** This is the single most important thing you can do for your health and weight loss. The best results can be achieved by combining a healthy diet with regular exercise.

• If weight loss with wheatgrass is something you're considering, it's important to discuss your plans with a doctor or registered dietitian first. They can tailor a program to your preferences and dietary requirements.

• Keep tabs on how well you're doing with your weight loss efforts so you can make any necessary adjustments. Keep in mind that a weight loss of 1-2 pounds per week is considered healthy.

• Wheatgrass may cause allergic reactions or gastrointestinal distress in a small percentage of the population. Pay attention to how your body responds, and cut back or stop using if necessary.

To sum up, wheatgrass can be an effective weight loss aid when combined with a healthy diet, regular exercise, and other healthy lifestyle choices. Never attempt to lose weight through diet alone; instead, talk to your doctor or a registered dietitian first.

CHAPTER THREE
Wheatgrass Aids Digestion

Wheatgrass is widely praised for its purported ability to aid digestion and reduce associated symptoms. While some people claim that wheatgrass has digestive benefits, it's important to note that scientific evidence supporting these claims is limited. Nonetheless, the following are some of the ways in which wheatgrass is thought to aid digestion:

1. Enzymes: The enzymes found in wheatgrass are thought to improve digestion and aid in the breakdown of food. Enzymes are essential for digestion because they help break down food into smaller, more absorbable pieces.

2. Wheatgrass has been linked to potential anti-inflammatory and detoxification properties due to the high chlorophyll content it contains. Inflammation and toxic buildup in the digestive tract can be alleviated by these properties.

3.Those who believe that consuming alkaline foods, such as wheatgrass, can help balance the body's pH levels and reduce acidity in the stomach and relieve symptoms of acid reflux or heartburn point to wheatgrass as an example.

4. Wheatgrass has a negligible amount of dietary fiber, which can aid in digestion and promote regular bowel movements. Constipation can be avoided and regular bowel movements can be encouraged thanks to fiber.

5. Some say that wheatgrass can help with detoxification by flushing out harmful substances like heavy metals and toxins from the digestive system, which could improve digestion and overall health.

Keep in mind that wheatgrass's ability to improve digestive health varies from person to person, and that the science behind these claims is weak. Wheatgrass may help some people with their gastrointestinal issues, while it may have no effect at all on others.

Here are a few things to remember if you want to use wheatgrass to aid digestion or alleviate digestive problems:

• If you've never tried wheatgrass before, ease into it by starting with a small amount. When first consuming wheatgrass, some people may experience stomach discomfort.

• Pay Attention to Your Reactions to WheatgrassBe aware of how your body reacts to wheatgrass. Do not continue using if you become nauseous or have stomach pain.

• A healthcare provider or gastroenterologist should be seen if persistent digestive problems or other health concerns are present. They can advise you on how to take care for your digestive system.

• You can improve your digestion by including wheatgrass in your diet, but it should be part of a well-rounded plan that also includes other nutrient-rich foods, fiber, and plenty of water.

- **Keep Yourself Well-hydrated:** Water helps digestion and is good for your health in general. When taking wheatgrass, it's important to drink enough of water.

Finally, additional scientific research is needed to validate the benefits of wheatgrass, which is often advertised as a digestive aid despite its effectiveness varying among individuals. Seek the advice of a medical expert if you are worried about your digestive system.

Wheatgrass and Physical Activity

Wheatgrass and exercise are two essential parts of a healthy lifestyle that can mutually benefit one another. The synergistic health benefits of exercise and wheatgrass are as follows:

• Wheatgrass' high nutrient content has led many to believe that it can be used as a natural energy booster. Wheatgrass, taken either before or after exercise, may help you push through your workouts with greater intensity.

• Wheatgrass can help supplement your diet, especially if you lead an active lifestyle, because to its high vitamin, mineral, and antioxidant content. These nutrients can help with muscle rehabilitation and overall health.

• Wheatgrass may aid in recovery by lowering exercise-induced inflammation and muscle pain due to its antioxidant and anti-inflammatory effects.

• Wheatgrass is a good source of water, which is essential for optimal performance during exercise. Wheatgrass is a great addition to your post-workout regimen and can help you feel more hydrated.

- Some people find that eating wheatgrass helps their digestion work better. Better nutrient absorption is essential for keeping your body fueled throughout activity, and a healthy digestive system can help with that.

- Some people believe that wheatgrass can help the body cleanse by removing toxins, but the evidence for this is scant. If you often partake in strenuous exercise or are exposed to high levels of environmental pollution, this may help you maintain your health and lessen the harmful burden on your body.

• Wheatgrass is low in calories and high in nutrients, making it a great complement to any diet aimed at weight maintenance or loss.

Here are some things to think about before adding wheatgrass to your workout routine:

• Wheatgrass can be taken either before or after exercise, depending on when you feel best. Some individuals take a wheatgrass shot first thing in the morning to get them going, while others use it as a recovery aid after a workout.

• If you've never tried wheatgrass before, ease into it by consuming only a small amount at first to see how your body reacts. When first adopting wheatgrass, some people may experience intestinal pain.

• Maintain an adequate water intake, since this will aid in both your performance and recovery after exercise. It's important to stay hydrated before, during, and after exercise.

• Wheatgrass has many health benefits, but it's best used as part of a varied, healthy diet that also includes lean meats, whole grains, fruits, and vegetables.

• Before making any major changes to your diet or exercise routine, you should talk to a doctor or qualified dietitian if you have any preexisting health conditions or dietary restrictions.

In conclusion, the synergistic effects of exercise and wheatgrass can help you stay healthy and happy. However, everyone react differently to wheatgrass, so it's crucial to pay attention to your body's reactions and talk to a doctor if you have any questions or concerns about adding wheatgrass to your workout routine.

CHAPTER FOUR
Keeping on Course

Maintaining focus on your health, fitness, personal growth, or any other set of goals can be difficult but ultimately rewarding. Some suggestions to keep you on track:

• Clearly define your objectives by writing them down. Make them specific, measurable, achievable, relevant, and time-bound (SMART). You now have something to shoot for.

• **Make a Strategy:** Think through what you need to do and how you need to do it in order to achieve your objectives. To avoid getting distracted, it helps to have a plan.

• Large objectives can be difficult to achieve all at once. Separate them into simpler steps that can be completed in one sitting. Enjoy the progress you've made so far.

• **Create a Schedule:** Make reaching your objectives a regular part of your workweek. The key to success is consistency. The more ingrained a behavior is, the simpler it is to keep doing.

• Share your goals with someone who can hold you accountable, such as a friend, family member, or mentor. You might also try keeping a journal or utilizing a smartphone app to monitor your development.

• Think on all the good things that will happen when you accomplish your goals, and do this regularly. Motivated and on course because of this, perhaps.

• Keep an Open Mind: Be ready to make changes to your strategy as needed. Being flexible is essential because of life's unpredictability.

• Maintain a Sense of Inspiration. Find role models in the form of books, podcasts, or people who have accomplished what you want to accomplish. Motivating examples of their achievements exist.

- **Self-compassion:** Be kind to yourself if you make mistakes or have trouble keeping up with your plans. Treat yourself kindly, and view failure as a stepping stone to success.

- Do not overextend yourself by taking on too many projects or responsibilities at once. Put your priorities first and work on just a few objectives at a time.

- **Time Management:** Learn to manage your time properly. Focus your efforts and energy on the activities that will get you the closest to your goals.

• Maintaining your physical and mental health is essential to succeeding in your goals. Make sure you're getting enough shut-eye, eating right, and working out consistently. Focus and drive can benefit from a healthy body and mind.

• **Mark Significant Milestones:** It is important to recognize and honor significant accomplishments. This can help you feel more accomplished and resolute in your efforts.

• Seek Help If you are having trouble maintaining your progress, you may want to talk to a therapist or counselor for guidance. They can aid in problem solving and the creation of effective plans for advancement.

• Keeping an optimistic outlook is essential. Keeping a positive outlook might give you the strength to persevere in the face of difficulty.

Keeping on track is an ongoing process, and it's natural to experience setbacks as you go. The capacity to stay focused on your goals and keep pushing forward in spite of setbacks is what really matters.

Meal Planning and Recipes

Making your own meal planning and recipes might help you eat well and stay on track with your weight loss goals. To assist you in getting going, here are some suggestions:

1. Consider Your Dietary Requirements

• Think about what you want to eat, what you can't eat, any food allergies you may have, and your overall health objectives. Recognizing your dietary requirements is the first step in developing a healthy eating strategy.

2. Make a plan to achieve your objectives:

• Set some dietary targets. Do you want to trim down, bulk up, get healthier generally, or control a chronic illness? Your diet plan should be based on your objectives.

3. Make a Meal Plan:

• Plan out how many meals and snacks you will eat daily. Common alternatives include three main meals and two snacks, although you can adjust this based on your needs and tastes.

4. Pick a Well-Rounding Diet:

• Try to eat items from all the different food categories on a regular basis. Fruits, vegetables, lean proteins, whole grains, and healthy fats are typical components of such a diet.

5. Figure Out How Many Calories You Need Each Day:

• Your daily calorie needs may need to be determined, depending on your objectives. If you want specific advice, you can utilize online calculators or talk to a dietician.

6. Develop Dishes:

• To begin, you should develop recipes that support your nutritional objectives. When feasible, try to use products that have been minimally processed. To maintain meal variety, try out new seasonings and cooking techniques.

7. Preparing Meals:

• Create a weekly or monthly menu plan. If you're looking to save time in the kitchen, try bulk cooking and planning your meals in advance. Include a wide range of foods and nutrients in your meal plan.

8. Dietary Restrictions:

• Mind your serving sizes. Weight gain is possible from any excessive eating, including nutritious meals. To help you keep your portion sizes in check, try using measuring cups, a food scale, or even just your eyes.

9. Have Snacks Ready:

• Eating nutritious snacks between meals helps keep you energized and prevent you from overindulging at mealtimes. Think ahead and stock up on healthy snacks like almonds, yogurt, and fruit.

10. Remember to drink plenty of water. In order to maintain good health, water is crucial. Prepare for the day by consuming enough water.

11. Keep a food journal or download a meal monitoring app to record what you eat each day. Maintaining accountability and making appropriate modifications will be facilitated by this.

12. Flexibility: - Allow some wiggle room in your diet. The unpredictability of life means that it's often necessary to make adjustments to your original plan.

13. Seek Expert Advice: - Talk to a registered dietitian or nutritionist if you have special dietary requirements, allergies, or health issues. They are able to give individualized advice and diet programs.

Breakfast:

• Eggs scrambled with vegetables

• Toasted whole grains

• A serving of fruit (bananas or berries, for example)

Lunch:

• A salad of grilled chicken or tofu over greens dressed with a vinaigrette

Snack:

• Honey-sweetened Greek yogurt
with a sprinkling of almonds

Dinner:

• Salmon or tofu stir-fried with
mixed veggies and baked

Pasta made with whole grains or
brown rice

Snack:

• Hummus and sliced veggies

Meal planning is an individual
process; your menu should be
tailored to your tastes and interests.
Make the required adjustments so

that it fits in with your plans and preferences.

CHAPTER FIVE
Controlling Food Losses

If you want to live a more eco-friendly and sustainable life, one of the first things you should do is find ways to waste less food. Environmental issues, such as greenhouse gas emissions and resource depletion, are exacerbated by food waste, which also has financial repercussions. If you want to waste less food, consider these suggestions.

1. Make a Meal Plan:

• Make a list of what you'll need to buy each week to create the meals you've planned. You'll be better able to control spending and get only what you require.

2. Spend Money Wisely

• Purchase foods with a longer shelf life and prioritize items that you know you will use beforc they expire. If you know you won't be able to use an item before it expires, avoid buying in bulk or taking advantage of "buy one, get one free" offers.

3. Verify the End Dates:

• Pay attention to expiration dates on food packaging. Use perishable things before they spoil, and make sure you can easily find them by sorting your pantry and fridge.

4. Follow the FIFO principle:

• Put the fresher food in the rear of the fridge and the older food in the front of the pantry. Using the older goods first is encouraged.

5. Maintaining food's freshness through proper storage is a must. Keep perishables fresh longer by storing them in the fridge (preferably in a crisper drawer) and using airtight containers and resealable bags.

6. Reading food labels correctly:

• Learn to read expiration dates on food packaging. The "Best Before" or "Use By" date indicates when the food will be at its peak freshness and safety. These "Sell By" dates are set with retailers in mind. You can tell if food is still edible by looking at it and smelling it.

7. Dietary Restrictions:

• When preparing and serving food, keep portion sizes in mind. This cuts down on food waste and prevents people from eating too much.

8. Leftovers:

• Don't throw away leftovers; find creative ways to use them. Make use of your fridge's leftovers by cooking up something delicious.

9. Composting:

Compost all of your kitchen leftovers and the bits of fruits and vegetables that won't be eaten. Reduce your impact on the environment and get nutrient-rich soil for your garden by composting.

10. Donate Extra Food: If you have extra canned goods or other non-perishable foods, think about giving them to a local food bank or charity.

11. If you have any perishable foods that you know you won't use before they spoil, it's best to freeze them. Many things can be frozen for later use, including fruits, vegetables, bread, and cooked meals.

12. Always take stock of what you have in your kitchen cabinets, fridge, and freezer. You may put long-forgotten goods to good use and prevent perishables from going to waste in this way.

13. Preserving Food Yourself: - Extend the shelf life of seasonal produce by learning how to can, pickle, or make jams and sauces.

14. If you have an abundance of food, whether it be homegrown or prepared, consider sharing it with others.

15. Learn as much as you can about the problems of food waste and environmental degradation. Knowing more will make you more interested in finding ways to cut down on waste.

Together, we can save money and save the planet by reducing food waste. Modifying your buying, cooking, and eating routines can greatly reduce your household's food waste.

Conclusion

Maintaining a healthy and balanced lifestyle involves a variety of factors, including nutrition, exercise, goal planning, and mindfulness. Important insights are as follows:

1. Good health begins in the kitchen with a varied intake of fresh produce, complete grains, lean proteins, and heart-healthy fats. To maintain your health, it's important to drink plenty of water and eat nutritious foods.

2. Working out on a consistent basis is crucial to the well-being of body and mind. Perform a range of activities, including aerobic, strength training, and stretching.

3. The secret to succeeding in many areas of life is to set goals that are both challenging and attainable. You'll be more focused and motivated if your goals are SMART (specific, measurable, achievable, relevant, and time-bound).

4. You can keep a positive outlook and deal with life's obstacles better via regular practice of mindfulness, self-compassion, and stress management skills.

5. Wheatgrass: Wheatgrass is a nutrient-dense food that can be added to your diet for potential health benefits like enhanced digestion, increased energy, and detoxification assistance. However, there is a wide range of scientific data backing its claims, and people have different reactions to it.

6. Minimizing food waste is a frugal and environmentally friendly action that helps people live more sustainably. Proper planning, storage, and conscientious consumption can help you reduce food waste.

Keep in mind that there is no one-size-fits-all path to wellness and equilibrium. It's crucial to modify these guidelines to fit your individual situation. Maintain a lifelong commitment to self-improvement and well-being, and see a doctor if you have any specific health issues or questions about your lifestyle choices.

THE END